Essential Oil Living

50+ Recipes for Everyday Life Using
Young Living® Essential Oils

Written & Compiled by

ALEXIS BAKER

TABLE OF CONTENTS

HELLO

Hi there! ! I'm so glad you're here :) My name is Alexis, and I'm delighted to share about one of my favorite things- essential oils!

In this booklet, you'll learn about oils in the "Introduction to Essential Oils" section which includes my personal experience just below. You'll also have an opportunity to learn about many of Young Living's® incredible essential oils and blends in the "About the Oils" section. The part I'm most excited about is giving you access to nearly 60 of my go-to DIY recipes I've created and collected over the years! Make sure to check out the links at the end too.

Thanks for picking up a copy of Essential Oil Living!
I hope you enjoy it and find joy in the journey!

MY STORY: WHY OILS?

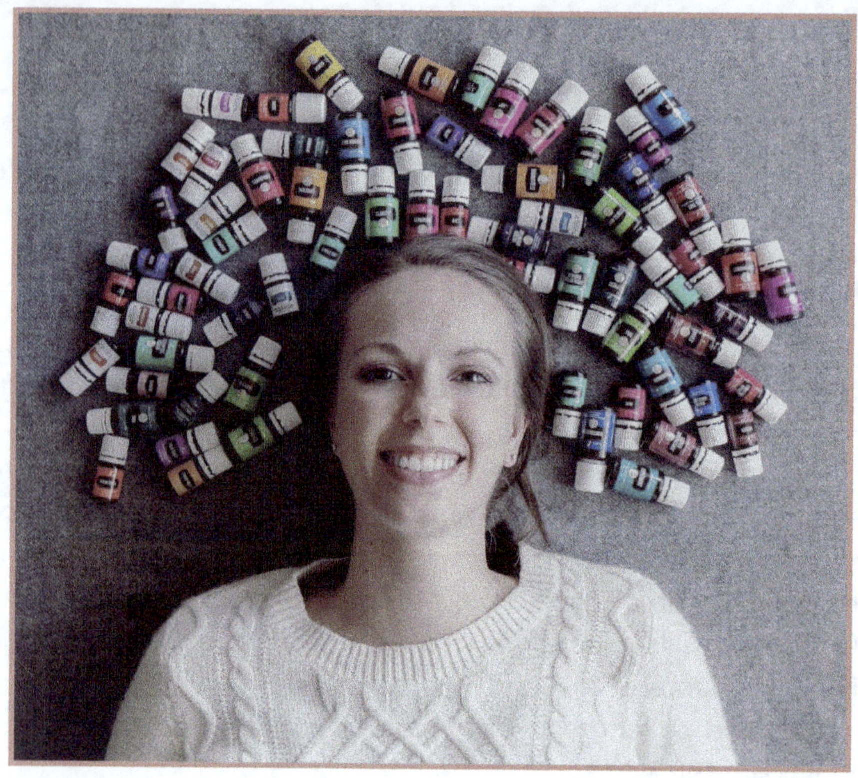

I first started hearing about essential oils in 2015, when a couple of friends mentioned them to me. My initial response: I was definitely skeptical, thought they were expensive, and didn't think I needed them. But as I began to hear more about oils and their incredible benefits, I had the thought that maybe I would at least try them one day. In February 2017, I launched my music therapy business, an endeavor I was very passionate about, but quickly realized there are a lot of ups and downs to starting and running a business!

I needed something to help me stay healthy by supporting my body physically, mentally and emotionally, but I wanted this something to be completely natural. So the following month, I decided to try essential oils and jumped all in by purchasing a starter kit from a company called Young Living®. I began using the oils every day, experimenting with different uses. I found they actually work because they were really helping me in a lot of ways!

The biggest impact oils have had on me is with my immune system. It's crazy to say, but I rarely get sick anymore. Oils have really helped strengthen my immune system. I'm also able to keep my stress and anxiety down. As a music therapist, I rely on my health to do my work. I depend heavily on my voice because every single music therapy session I do involves singing, and I lead multiple MT groups every week. I have to be functioning well or else I can't work. Back in 2014, I began to get sick constantly...colds, flus, even strep throat. This went on for a few years and was not fun! Since beginning to use oils consistently however, I've noticed I get sick much less each year. My immune system has gotten stronger over time from consistent use of oils, and I can better handle the daily stresses of running a business and the physical tolls of being a music therapist. I also work with older adults who tend to have weakened immune systems and health issues, so it's critical for me to be healthy around them. Essential oils have helped me with more than just my immune function though... things like getting better sleep, taking care of my skin, energy, mood, emotions, and reducing stress. Let's dive in and learn more!

TOXINS, TOXINS EVERYWHERE

Environmental toxins are pretty much everywhere.
Chemicals are in soaps, shampoos, makeup, air fresheners,
cleaning products, even our furniture and more.

Consider these statistics:

- ⚠ As of 2009, the EU has banned 1,328 chemicals, while
  the US has only ever banned 30.
- ⚠ There are roughly 87,000 chemicals registered in the
  US. Only 10-15% of those have ever been tested for
  potential health effects.
- ⚠ The average person applies 300 chemicals to their
  body every day. About 80 of those are applied before
  breakfast.

Some of the harmful ingredients found in products include:

- o Bismuth
- o Synthetic colors
- o Fragrance
- o Parabens
- o Talc
- o Lead
- o Mercury
- o SLS (sodium laurel sulfate)
- o Phthalates

Negative effects of these harmful chemicals can include headaches, dermatitis, allergic reactions, respiratory distress, bioaccumulation, damage to immune system, and more.

In studies, many of these harmful chemicals have been linked to cancer, birth defects, reproductive issues, hyperactivity, asthma, and more.

While this may be scary and should be cause for alarm, there are so many ways we can eliminate toxic products and switch to safe, natural ones decreasing the amount of toxins we expose our bodies to on a daily basis. We just need to be intentional about it.

WHAT ARE ESSENTIAL OILS?

Essential oils are the most powerful part of plants known as the lifeblood. They protect them from disease, provide nutrients and help keep them healthy, strong and functioning at their best. They're distilled from various parts of plants such as the flowers, leaves or roots. Essential oils were mankind's first medicine! They've existed for thousands of years and only recently "rediscovered." Some of the oldest cultures on earth used essential oils. Today, they're still used to promote health in the body physically, mentally, spiritually and emotionally. Oils are very complex, containing hundreds of different organic chemical compounds. The molecules that make up essential oils are so tiny they can pass through the wall of every single cell in the body, allowing them to support and aid cells at the most fundamental levels of your body. (There are actually 40 million trillion molecules in one drop of essential oil!) They do things like clean out receptor sites and create conditions that unfriendly virus and bacteria can't survive. Basically, essential oils work in different ways to balance and restore the body to harmony.

SUPPORTING YOUR BODY'S SYSTEMS NATURALLY WITH ESSENTIAL OILS

Essential oils can aid in the function of every single system of the body at a cellular level. From supporting digestion to boosting the immune system, there's literally an oil to assist all the body's functions in one way or another.

Young Living®'s premium essential oils can:

- reach every cell in your body within 20 minutes when applied topically
- be absorbed through the skin and into the bloodstream
- bypass digestion when inhaled or used topically
- eliminate toxins from the body
- cross the blood-brain barrier
- affect emotions via the limbic system of your brain when inhaled
- clean receptor sites in the brain

- relax and clear the mind
- act as powerful antioxidants
- remove toxins in the air

CHOOSING THE RIGHT GRADE

Did you know that not all essential oils are created equal? That's right - there may be up to 4 different categories or "grades" that all oils fall into: Grade A, B, C and D. It's vitally important to choose and use oils that are Grade A only. Here's why:

- Grade A oils are made from organically grown plants and distilled at low temperatures. Overheating an oil can destroy it, so the distillation process must take place at correct temperatures. These oils are considered pure and therapeutic quality.
- Grade B oils are considered food grade; however, they may contain synthetics such as pesticides, fertilizers, chemical extenders and carrier oils.
- Grade C are categorized as perfume oils, frequently include impure substances, and are commonly mixed with chemicals. These oils often employ solvents, like hexane, to maximize the amount of oil obtained from each harvest. These solvents can be carcinogenic and are present in numerous oils available in stores. Additionally, Grade C oils may be diluted with alcohol, typically comprising 80-95% of the final product.

Grade D can be considered "floral water." It refers to a type of fragrance that is primarily aromatic and is typically obtained as a byproduct during the distillation process of Grade A oils. Once all the oil has been extracted, the remaining waste water is sold to companies. These companies then fill around 5 percent of the bottle with this residual floral water and fill the remainder with carrier oils like coconut oil and grape seed oil, labeling it as "pure."

Many different factors affect the quality of essential oils. Grade B, C and D oils might smell nice and produce a pleasant experience, but there are a few reasons why it's a good idea to opt for Grade A oils only. For example, with Grade B, C and D oils, you may be wasting money on an inferior product, the oils lack the full benefits, and using them could actually be detrimental or harmful to your body. Before purchasing oils, I would advise thorough research into the type and brand, considering how the company creates its oils: Do they maintain control over the entire process or only part of it? Do they grow their own plants or source them? Do they distill their own oils or source them? Do they test every batch and use third party testing? There are many points along the way in the production process that an oil could lose its purity.

APPLICATION AND METHODS OF USE

Tests have shown essential oils reach the heart, liver and thyroid in 3 seconds when inhaled. When applied topically, they were found in the bloodstream in 26 seconds. Twenty minutes after application, they reach every cell in the body. Expulsion of essential oils takes 3-6 hours in a normal, healthy body.

There are 3 main ways to use essential oils: topically, aromatically and internally. I would suggest these methods only if you're certain you have absolutely pure oils.

TOPICAL USE

As you may already be aware, our skin is our largest organ, and it absorbs roughly 80% of what we put on it. Direct application onto the skin is one of the easiest ways to use essential oils because the molecules then pass through our cell walls. Some essential oils can be applied neat (undiluted) while dilution (combining with a carrier oil) is recommended with others. Always dilute when using essential oils with kiddos. Some examples of carrier oils include fractionated coconut oil, grape seed oil, vitamin E oil, sweet almond oil and jojoba oil. The carrier oil you use is more a matter of preference or whether you're concerned about the comedogenic rating of it. The bottoms of your feet, insides of your wrists, and the back of your neck are generally good spots to apply oils topically.

AROMATIC USE

Aromatic use of essential oils is believed to be the most effective method because the molecules don't have to pass through the skin or the digestive system. When oils are inhaled, they immediately enter the olfactory system. The sense of smell is more powerful than we realize as it's the only sense that has a direct connection to the brain. The olfactory system directly affects the limbic system, which deals with emotions, memories, arousal and motivation.

Here are several methods for aromatic use of oils:

1. Choose an oil that either appeals to you or you know you need in that moment and breathe in straight from the bottle.
2. Inhale with intention by placing a couple drops in your palms, rubbing your hands together, then cupping them over your mouth and nose while inhaling deeply.
3. Diffusing oils can be a very uplifting and refreshing experience. Using a diffuser is the perfect way to instantly improve your living or work environment. Some oils can purify the air by removing toxins and neutralizing bad odors. Diffusing oils can also help with mood regulation.
4. Try using diffuser jewelry, such as a necklace or bracelet.
5. Take a bath with Epsom salt and oils. Add 3-6 drops oil of choice to one cup Epsom salt. You'll get both the aromatic and topical benefits simultaneously.

INTERNAL USE

The Food and Drug Administration (FDA) classifies certain essential oils as GRAS (generally recognized as safe) for consumption. Young Living® is the only company that has oils specifically labeled for internal or dietary use. They worked directly with the FDA to ensure GRAS and even came up with unique labeling to meet regulations and help consumers know which oils are safe for ingestion. I don't recommend consuming oils from any other brand than Young Living®—they're the only company with this approval. Young Living® bottles with white labeling and the "Vitality™" banner just below the oil name are safe to ingest. Try these methods for internal or dietary use:

1. Add a couple drops to your water, tea, smoothie or other beverage.
2. Make your own supplement by adding 3-8 drops of oil to an empty veggie capsule, then filling the rest with olive or avocado oil.
3. Try cooking or baking with them—you can add them to salad dressings, marinades, sauces and more!

WHY YOUNG LIVING®?

Essential oils are the type of product where you generally get what you pay for. One of the many reasons I chose and love the Young Living® brand is their Seed to Seal® process and promise. Young Living® is all about transparency. They can guarantee the purity of their oils because they control the entire production from the farm to your home. You can visit seedtoseal.com for more information.

Young Living® is one of the largest and most trusted essential oil company in the world. They have been around for over 25 years leading the essential oil industry with their uncompromised standards of quality and purity. They have a huge range of oils along with hundreds of other wellness and personal care products.

Young Living'®s products are unparalleled. They are high quality and support a more toxin-free lifestyle. We've been loyal Young Living® members since 2017 because we have peace of mind ordering from them over and over. If you want to live a more toxin-free life, essential oils are a great place to start. Essential oils are a like bridge to natural living. They can help you swap out the products containing harmful, toxic ingredients for more natural, plant-based ones, but the choice is up to you! Each person is the gatekeeper to their own home.

To wrap up this introduction to essential oils, I want to pass along a challenge to you. It's called the "Three-Cabinet Challenge." If you're at home, choose 3 cabinets and pull a few products out from each. Look in your laundry room, under your kitchen sink and in your bathroom. Read the ingredients that are in the products you're using to clean your home, care for your body or ingest. If you're not sure what an ingredient is or whether it's safe, type the word into Google with the words "dangers of" in front of it and do a little research.

Why oils? Because every oil you use is a potentially harmful chemical you're not using. We can't control all of the toxins we're exposed to, but we can decide what we allow in our homes. It's up to you to make a better choice today and start using essential oils rather than products toxic to our health and wellness. You can literally replace all your personal care and home cleaning products with oil-infused products. Just start with one small step at a time.

STARTING YOUR OIL JOURNEY

The question I probably get the most is "What oils should I purchase to get started?" While it's a challenge to narrow it down because there truly are so many valuable oils, these dozen are a great place to start. This list is of course subjective, but these oils are all amazing and will help build your health up over the long run while also addressing everyday issues like stress, upset stomach and sleep. In addition, these oils will help anyone create a more toxin-free home and lifestyle. You can learn more about these 12 oils and others in the "About the Oils" section.

1. Lemon
2. Lavender
3. Peppermint
4. Thieves®
5. Stress Away™
6. Eucalyptus
7. Panaway™
8. Lemongrass
9. Frankincense
10. Cedarwood
11. Purification®
12. Christmas Spirit™

SAFETY

It's important go over safety when talking about essential oils, so here are some tips and guidelines:

- Certain oils are photosensitive, meaning you don't want to apply them and then be out in direct sunlight because it can lead to skin burns. These are mostly the citrus oils, like grapefruit and lemon. Wait at least 12 hours before going in direct sunlight if you 've applied a photosensitive oil.

- Dilution is recommended for some oils, especially the more "hot" or "spicy" oils such as Thieves® or peppermint. You should always dilute when using oils with kids.

- For newborns, the strength of the smell of the oil can, in rare cases, lead to respiratory issues. So, when holding them, make sure you aren't wearing strong-smelling oils such as eucalyptus, basil, juniper, peppermint, hyssop and wintergreen. It is not recommended to use oils topically on babies under 6 months, but diffusing is welcome.

- Even though it's common sense, keep oils out of eyes, ears and other sensitive areas. If you ever get them in your eye, wash out with a carrier oil, not water. Oil and water don't mix, but a carrier oil will help dilute and wash it away.

- A general rule is to start low and go slow: A little goes a long way, so start with fewer drops and space out use.
- Put citrus oils in glass or stainless steel only when mixing with a beverage—not plastic.
- Store oils in a cool, dark place. Young Living® oils actually never expire as long as they're properly stored.

DISCLAIMER

The information about essential oils provided in this booklet does not intend to treat, cure, diagnose, or prevent any diseases or illnesses. If you believe you have a medical condition, it is strongly recommended that you consult a qualified healthcare professional. Before making changes to your current health routine, it is advisable to seek guidance from your healthcare provider. The suggestions mentioned in this booklet are intended for use with pure, therapeutic-grade essential oils that are appropriately labeled for such use. It should be understood that the publisher and authors are not responsible for any misunderstandings or misuse of the information provided in this booklet.

Essential oil rollers can be used for many different purposes—to aid in better sleep, relaxation, emotional support, boost the immune system and more—not to mention, they can make a great perfume. Enjoy this collection of 14 roller recipes!

RELAX

- o 10ml roller bottle
- o 20 drops Stress Away™
- o 10 drops Lavender
- o 10 drops Northern Lights Black Spruce
- o 10 drops Sacred Frankincense
- o Fractionated coconut oil (or carrier oil of choice)

Add essential oil drops to the bottle, then top with carrier oil. Insert the roller top. Apply to wrists, bottoms of feet or back of neck as needed.

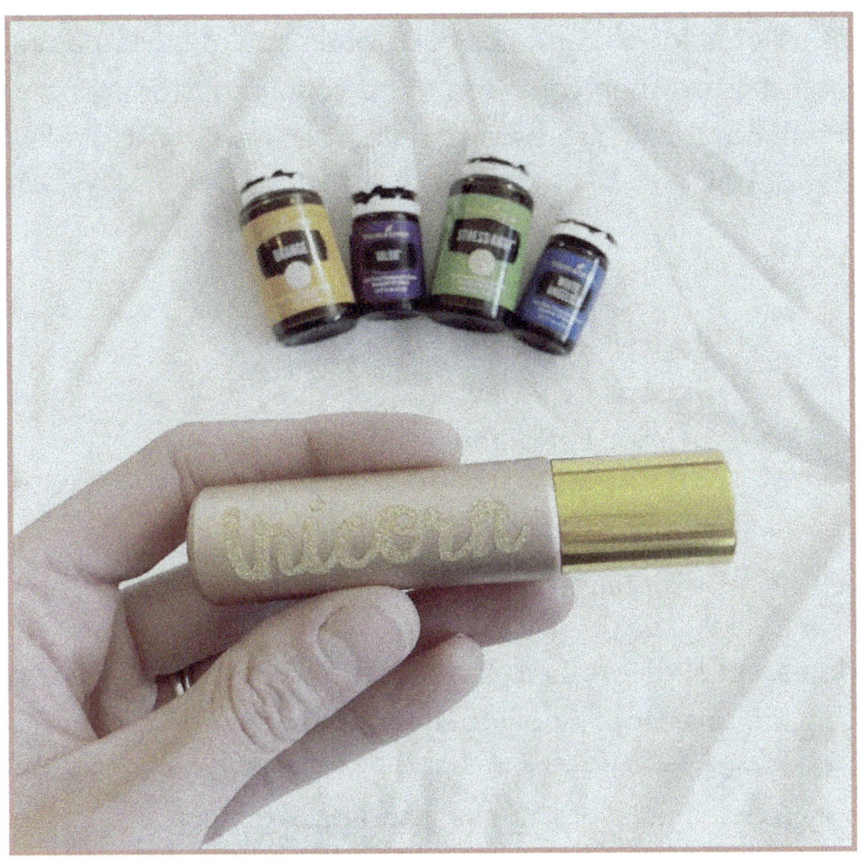

UNICORN

- o   10ml roller bottle
- o   15 drops Valor®
- o   15 drops White Angelica™
- o   15 drops Stress Away™
- o   15 drops Orange or Lime
- o   Fractionated coconut oil (or carrier oil of choice)

Add essential oil drops to the bottle, then top with carrier oil. Insert the roller top. Apply to wrists, bottoms of feet or back of neck as needed.

This roller is for big emotions like when you're having a really tough day, or when you need to be courageous or brave with something. It can also be a perfume because it just smells so dang good!

TENSION TAMER

- o 10ml roller bottle
- o 15 drops Panaway™
- o 15 drops Peppermint
- o 15 drops Frankincense
- o 15 drops Lavender
- o Fractionated coconut oil (or carrier oil of choice)

Add essential oil drops to the bottle, then top with carrier oil. Insert the roller top. Apply to areas of concern—rub over tight or sore muscles, areas with aches or pain; for head tension, apply to hairline (avoiding eyes) and back of neck.

CHILL OUT

- o 5ml roller bottle
- o 15 drops Stress Away™
- o 15 drops Lavender
- o Fractionated coconut oil (or carrier oil of choice)

Add essential oil drops to the bottle, then top with coconut oil. Insert the roller top. Apply to wrists, bottoms of feet or back of neck as needed.

Tip: Reuse your old 5ml essential oil bottles to make rollers by cleaning them and then using the AromaGlide™ Roller Fitments from Young Living®. Here are the steps I use to remove the labels and thoroughly clean the bottles:

1. Slowly peel labels off.
2. Soak in hot, soapy water and scrub the outside of the bottles.
3. Rinse and let air dry.
4. Put 5-6 drops of lemon essential oil on a cotton pad and use it to get any remaining label residue off.
5. Run bottles through the dishwasher facing down and let air dry.

CALM

- o 5ml roller bottle
- o 15 drops Peace & Calming®
- o 15 drops Lavender
- o Fractionated coconut oil (or carrier oil of choice)

Add essential oil drops to the bottle, then top with coconut oil. Insert the roller top. Apply to wrists, bottoms of feet or back of neck as needed.

LIGHTS OUT

- o   10ml roller bottle
- o   15 drops Lavender
- o   15 drops Cedarwood
- o   15 drops Frankincense
- o   15 drops Vetiver
- o   Fractionated coconut oil (or carrier oil of choice)

Add essential oil drops to the bottle, then top with carrier oil. Insert the roller top. Apply to wrists, bottoms of feet or back of neck as needed at bedtime. (Recipe adapted from *The EO Bar* app.)

SWEET DREAMS

- o   10ml roller bottle
- o   20 drops Bergamot
- o   20 drops Lavender
- o   20 drops Cedarwood
- o   Fractionated coconut oil (or carrier oil of choice)

Add essential oil drops to the bottle, then top with coconut oil. Insert the roller top. Apply to wrists, bottoms of feet or back of neck as needed at bedtime.

HAPPY

- o   10ml roller bottle
- o   15 drops Stress Away™
- o   15 drops Lemon
- o   10 drops Joy™
- o   10 drops Valor®
- o   Fractionated coconut oil (or carrier oil of choice)

Add essential oil drops to the bottle, then top with coconut oil. Insert the roller top. Apply to wrists, bottoms of feet or back of neck as needed.

CITRUS BLISS

- o   5ml roller bottle
- o   15 drops Stress Away™
- o   15 drops Citrus Fresh™
- o   Fractionated coconut oil (or carrier oil of choice)

Add essential oil drops to the bottle, then top with coconut oil. Insert the roller top. Apply to wrists, bottoms of feet or back of neck as needed.

IMMUNE BOOSTER

- o 10 ml roller bottle
- o 20 drops Frankincense
- o 20 drops Lemon
- o 20 drops Thieves®
- o Fractionated coconut oil (or carrier oil of choice)

Add essential oil drops to the bottle, then top with coconut oil. Insert the roller top. Apply to spine, bottoms of feet or back of neck as needed.

How the Thieves® blend got its name: It's said the name of this oil blend was inspired by legends of four 15th-century French thieves who formulated a special aromatic combination composed of rosemary, clove and several other botanicals. They used this blend to protect themselves from illness while robbing from dead bodies as well as those sick and dying.

CHILL BABY

- o 5ml roller bottle
- o 10 drops Gentle Baby™
- o Fractionated coconut oil (or carrier oil of choice)

Add essential oil drops to the bottle, then top with carrier oil. Insert the roller top. Apply to bottoms of feet. This roller is great for helping little ones calm down when they 're fussy, or it can be used as part of nap/bedtime routine.

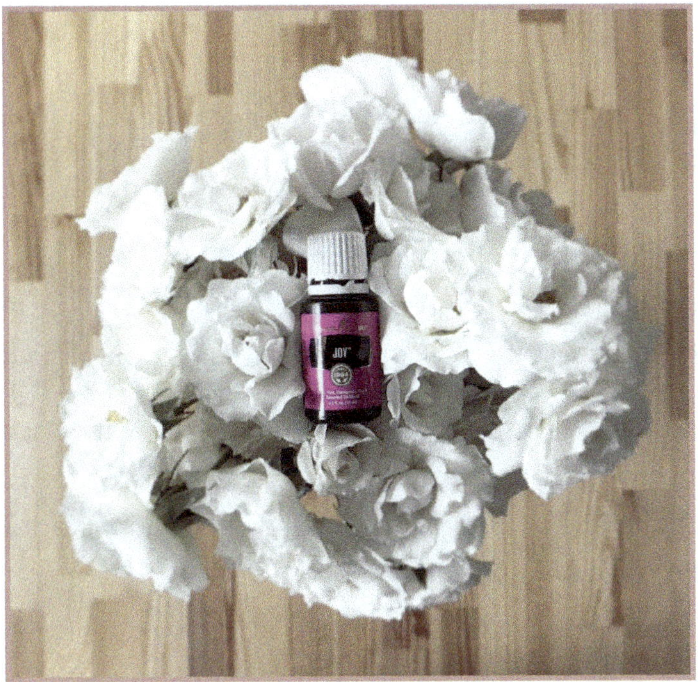

STARDUST

- o   10ml roller bottle
- o   10 drops Lavender
- o   10 drops Valor®
- o   10 drops Stress Away™
- o   10 drops Joy™
- o   10 drops Vetiver
- o   Fractionated coconut oil (or carrier oil of choice)

Add essential oil drops to the bottle, then top with coconut oil. Insert the roller top. Apply to spine, bottoms of feet or back of neck as needed. (Recipe originally found on Instagram from Aubrey Kinch: @something.essential)

RAINBOW

- o   10ml roller bottle
- o   15 drops Sacred Mountain™
- o   15 drops Bergamot
- o   10 drops Stress Away™
- o   8 drops Idaho Blue Spruce
- o   8 drops Tangerine
- o   Fractionated coconut oil (or carrier oil of choice)

Add essential oil drops to the bottle, then top with coconut oil. Insert the roller top. Apply to spine, bottoms of feet or back of neck as needed. (Recipe originally found on Instagram from Kristin Fox: @oilyroseessentials)

TRANQUIL*

- o   10ml roller bottle
- o   30 drops Lavender
- o   25 drops Cedarwood
- o   15 drops Roman Chamomile
- o   Fractionated coconut oil (or carrier oil of choice)

Add essential oil drops to the bottle, then top with coconut oil. Insert the roller top. Apply to wrists, bottoms of feet or back of neck as needed.

*This is a Young Living® roller blend copycat recipe.

DIFFUSER BOMBS

As I mentioned earlier, diffusing oils can be a very uplifting and refreshing experience. Using a diffuser is the perfect way to instantly improve your living or work environment. I hope you enjoy this collection of 14 seasonal diffuser recipes!

ROOM REFRESH (SPRING)

- o   4 drops Lemon
- o   4 drops Lavender
- o   2 drops Peppermint

LEMON GROVE (SPRING)

- o   3 drops Jade Lemon
- o   2 drops Lemon
- o   2 drops Ylang Ylang
- o   2 drops Eucalyptus Globulus
- o   2 drops Spearmint

SPRING CLEAN (SPRING)

- o   3 drops Lemon
- o   3 drops Lime
- o   2 drops Lavender
- o   2 drops Rosemary

SPRING BREEZE (SPRING)

- o   4 drops Grapefruit
- o   3 drops Cedarwood
- o   3 drops Rosemary
- o   2 drops Eucalyptus

ANTHROPOLOGIE (SUMMER)

- o   3 drops Lime
- o   3 drops Tangerine
- o   3 drops Grapefruit
- o   3 drops Valor®

UNICORN (SUMMER)

- o   3 drops Valor®
- o   3 drops White Angelica™
- o   3 drops Stress Away™
- o   3 drops Lime

PINK LEMONADE (SUMMER)

- o   5 drops Lemon
- o   5 drops Valor®

PUMPKIN SPICE (FALL/WINTER)

- o   4 drops Clove
- o   3 drops Orange
- o   2 drops Nutmeg
- o   2 drops Cinnamon Bark

IMMUNE BOOSTER (FALL/WINTER)

- o   4 drops Thieves®
- o   4 drops Lemon
- o   4 drops Frankincense

MARSHMALLOW (FALL/WINTER)

- o   4 drops Nutmeg
- o   4 drops Cinnamon Bark
- o   4 drops Ylang Ylang
- o   2 drops Bergamot
- o   3 drops Stress Away™

SWEATER WEATHER (FALL/WINTER)

- o   5 drops Vanilla
- o   4 drops Christmas Spirit™
- o   3 drops Northern Lights Black Spruce

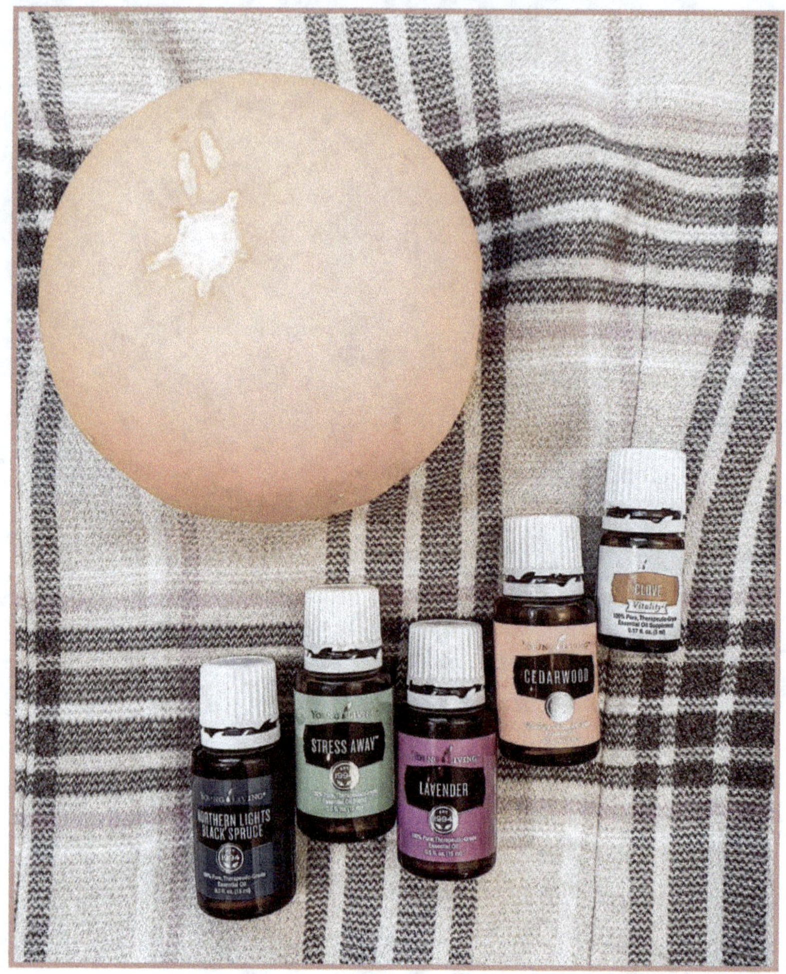

COZY BLANKET (FALL/WINTER)

- 5 drops Northern Lights Black Spruce
- 3 drops Stress Away™
- 2 drops Cedarwood
- 2 drops Lavender
- 2 drops Clove

SPICED CINNAMON (FALL/WINTER)

- o 5 drops Stress Away™
- o 4 drops Cinnamon Bark
- o 2 drops Clove

FOCUS (YEAR-ROUND)

- o 4 drops Lemon
- o 3 drops Frankincense
- o 2 drops Peppermint

SPRAYS

From room sprays to a calming pillow spray to protecting yourself against pesky insects, using essential oils in sprays not only makes them smell amazing but they can also replace harmful chemicals many conventional products contain. Enjoy this collection of 5 spray bottle recipes!

ROOM REFRESH SPRAY

- o   4 oz. glass fine mist spray bottle
- o   20 drops Lavender
- o   20 drops Eucalyptus Radiata
- o   Distilled water
- o   Witch hazel

Add essential oil drops to the bottle. Fill 2/3 of the bottle with water and remaining 1/3 with witch hazel. Shake gently before each use. Spray around the room or mist over linens, couch or bed. Can be used as a car spray as well. Try subbing lavender and eucalyptus for other oils such as Christmas Spirit™.

BATHROOM DEODORIZER SPRAY

- o   4 oz. glass fine mist spray bottle
- o   25 drops Purification®
- o   15 drops Lemon
- o   Distilled water
- o   Witch hazel

Add essential oil drops to the bottle, fill 2/3 of the bottle with water and remaining 1/3 with hazel. Shake gently before each use. Spray 3-4 times around the room or on your towel or bathmat.

LINEN SPRAY

- o   2 oz. glass fine mist spray bottle
- o   15 drops Calm™
- o   10 drops Lavender
- o   Distilled water
- o   Witch hazel

Add essential oil drops to the bottle. Fill 2/3 of the bottle with water and remaining 1/3 with witch hazel. Shake gently before each use. Mist over lines, bedding, and pillows.

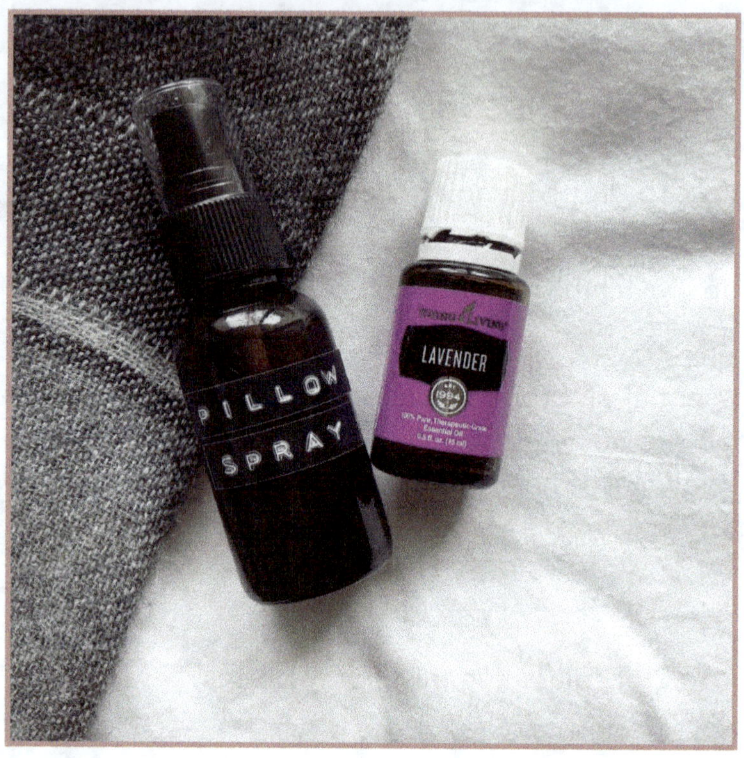

CALMING PILLOW SPRAY

- o   2 oz. glass fine mist spray bottle
- o   15 drops Lavender
- o   5 drops Stress Away™
- o   Distilled water
- o   Witch hazel

Add essential oil drops to the bottle. Fill 2/3 of the bottle with water and remaining 1/3 with witch hazel. Shake gently before each use. Mist over pillow and bedding.

PEST PROTECTION SPRAY

- o 4 oz. glass fine mist spray bottle
- o 15 drops Citronella
- o 10 drops Peppermint
- o 10 drops Lavender
- o 10 drops Purification®
- o Distilled water
- o Alcohol-free witch hazel

Add essential oil drops to the bottle. Fill 2/3 of the bottle with water and remaining 1/3 with witch hazel. Shake gently before each use. Mist over body and clothing when outdoors.

PERSONAL CARE & BEAUTY

This is one of my favorite sections because the recipes are so practical! I've been using many of these recipes for years now and have shared them with others who LOVE them too. I hope you enjoy this collection of 12 personal care and beauty recipes.

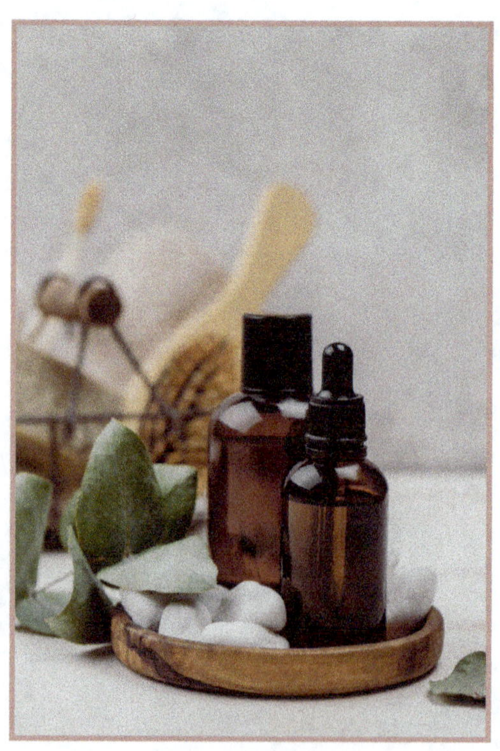

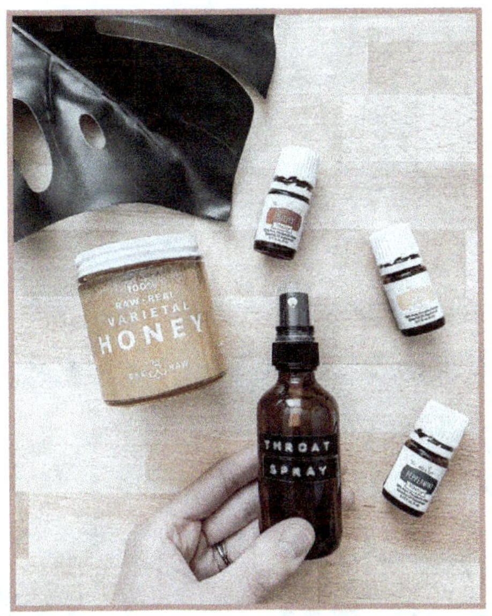

THROAT SPRAY

- o   2 oz. glass fine mist spray bottle
- o   1 ½ oz. purified water
- o   10 drops Thieves® Vitality™
- o   5 drops Peppermint Vitality™
- o   5 drops Lemon Vitality™
- o   1 tsp. Honey

Add essential oil drops to the bottle. Heat water up so honey will dissolve and mix in thoroughly. Let cool, then pour into the spray bottle and give it a good shake!

Tip: If you're a singer like me, this spray is great for vocal health. When your voice feels tired or strained, use this spray. If you're dealing with a scratchy or sore throat, use this spray.

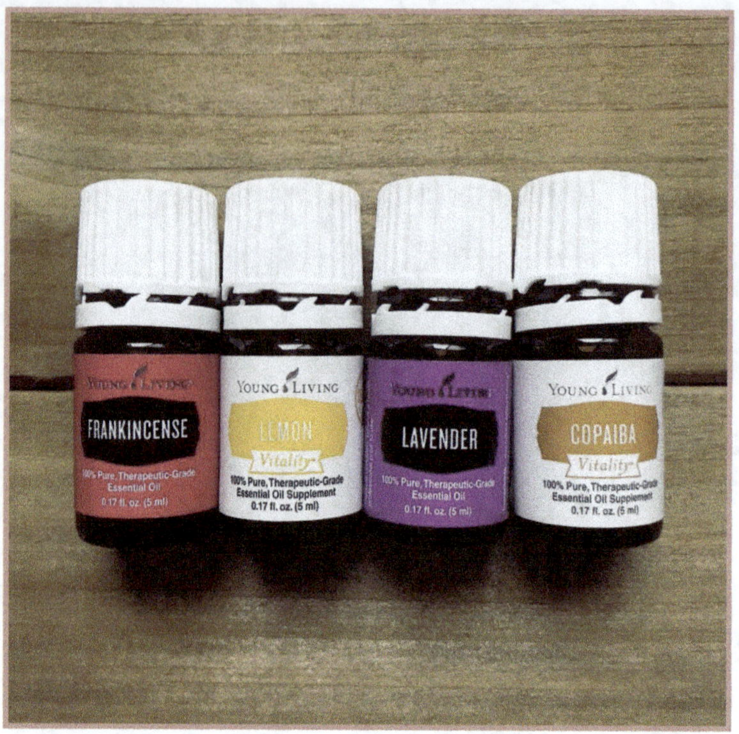

UNDER-EYE SERUM

- o   5ml roller bottle
- o   10 drops Frankincense
- o   10 drops Lemon
- o   10 drops Lavender
- o   10 drops Copaiba
- o   Castor oil (or carrier oil of choice)

Add essential oil drops to the bottle, then top with carrier oil. Insert the roller top. Gently apply to the skin under eyes just before bed, taking care to avoid direct contact with eyes.

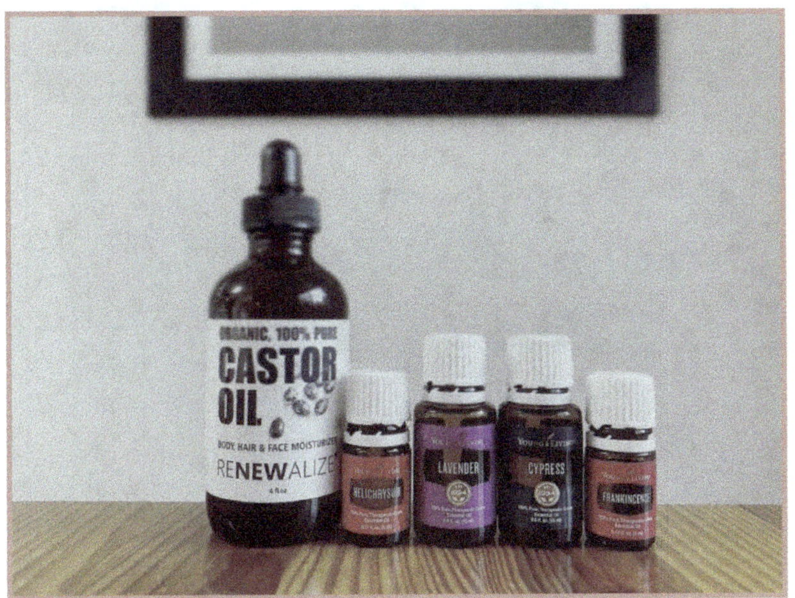

SCAR ROLLER

- o   5ml roller bottled
- o   10 drops Lavender
- o   10 drops Frankincense
- o   10 drops Helichrysum
- o   10 drops Cypress
- o   Castor oil (or carrier oil of choice)

Add essential oil drops to the bottle, then top with carrier oil. Insert the roller top. Apply to scars on face or other areas of the body. Gently massage in after application.

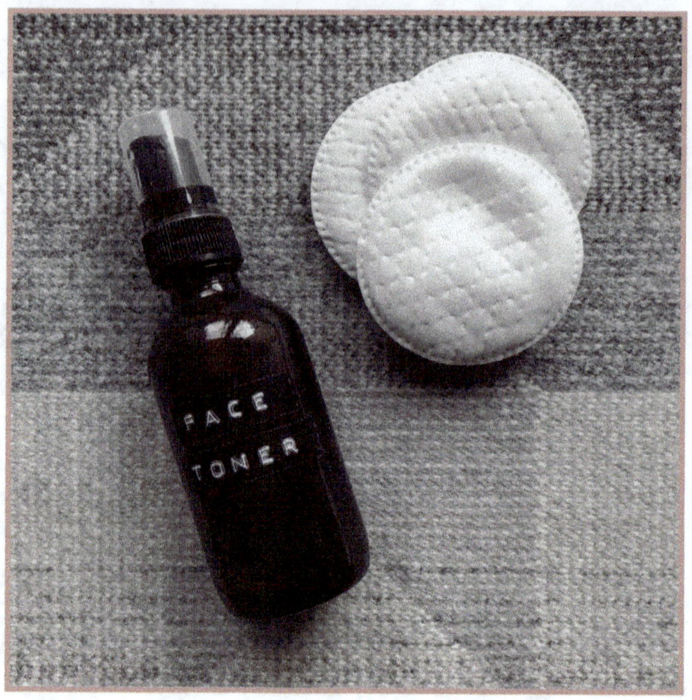

FACE TONER

- o 2 oz. glass fine mist spray bottle
- o 4 drops Lavender
- o 4 drops Frankincense
- o 3 drops Cedarwood
- o 3 drops Orange
- o 2 drops Peppermint
- o 2 drops Blue tansy (optional)
- o Alcohol-free witch hazel

Add essential oil drops to the bottle and top with witch hazel. Shake gently before each use. Can either spritz directly onto face (with eyes closed) or onto a cotton round.

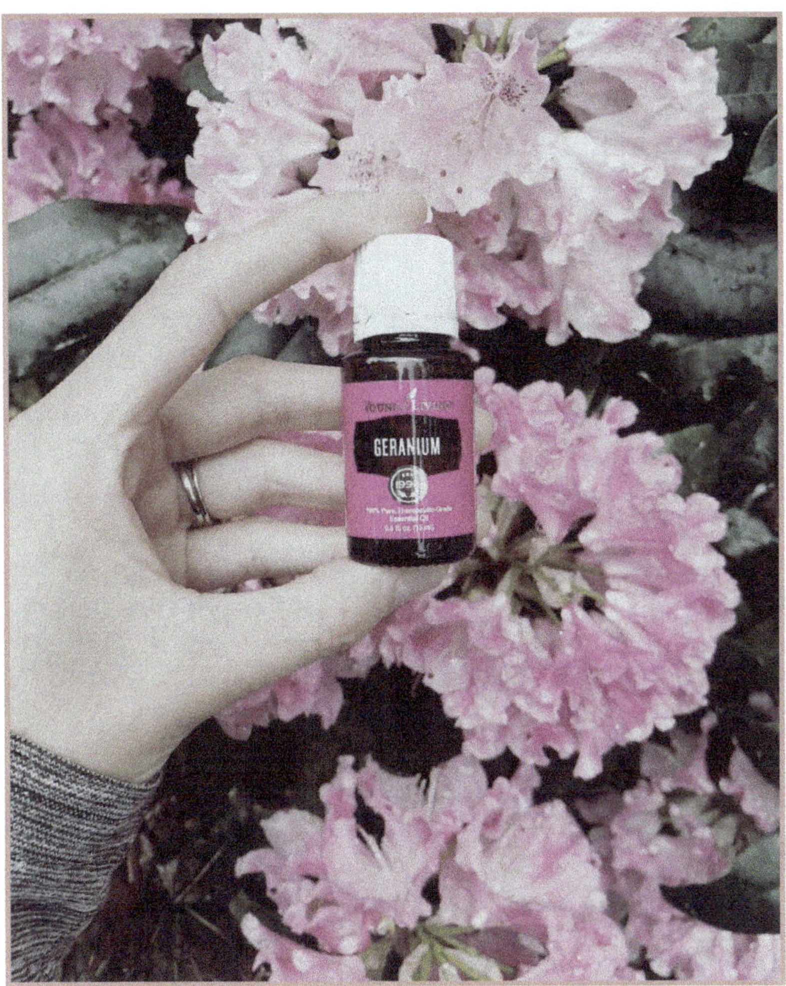

MERMAID HAIR

- o 4 oz. glass fine mist spray bottle
- o 15 drops Lavender
- o 15 drops Cedarwood
- o 15 drops Rosemary
- o 10 drops Geranium (optional)
- o Alcohol-free witch hazel

Add essential oil drops to the bottle, top with witch hazel. Shake gently before each use. Spritz on your hair at the roots, wet or dry.

HAPPY BODY MIST

- o 2 oz. glass fine mist spray bottle
- o 10 drops Joy™
- o 10 drops Orange
- o Alcohol-free witch hazel
- o Distilled water

Add essential oil drops to the bottle. Fill 2/3 of the bottle with water and remaining 1/3 with witch hazel. Shake gently before each use. Mist over body.

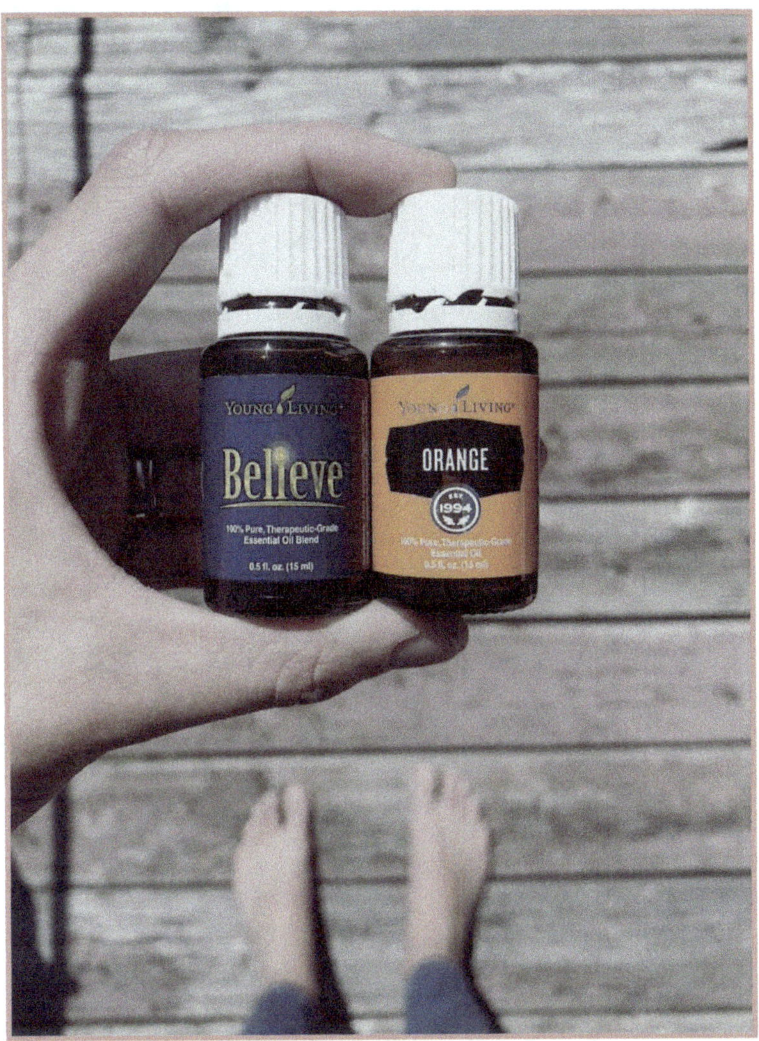

BELIEVE BODY MIST

- o   2 oz. glass fine mist spray bottle
- o   10 drops Believe™
- o   10 drops Orange
- o   Alcohol-free witch hazel
- o   Distilled water

Add essential oil drops to the bottle. Fill 2/3 of the bottle with water and remaining 1/3 with witch hazel. Shake gently before each use. Mist over body.

STRESS LESS BODY MIST

- o   2 oz. glass fine mist spray bottle
- o   20 drops Stress Away™
- o   Alcohol-free witch hazel
- o   Distilled water

Add essential oil drops to the bottle. Fill 2/3 of the bottle with water and remaining 1/3 with witch hazel. Shake gently before each use. Mist over body.

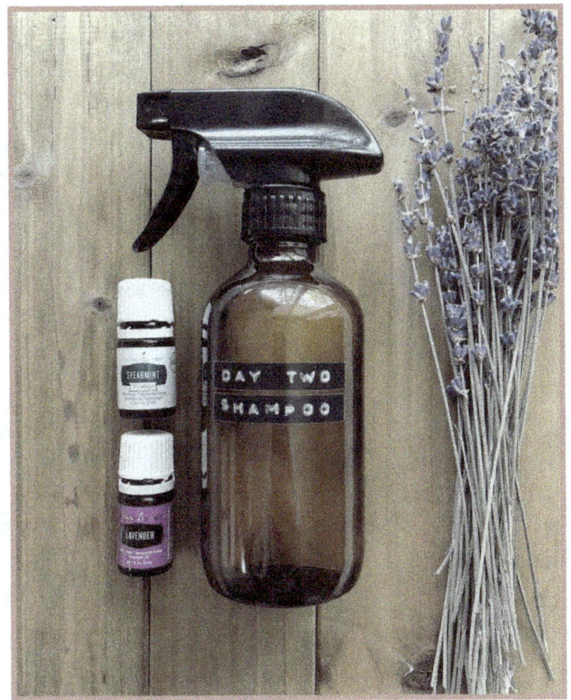

DAY TWO SHAMPOO

- o 8 oz. glass spray bottle
- o 1 cup warm distilled water
- o ¼ cup arrowroot powder
- o ¼ cup alcohol-free witch hazel
- o 20 drops Lavender
- o 20 drops Spearmint

Mix everything together in the bottle and shake well. Separation will occur, so shake well before each use. Spray on roots or oily parts of hair. Let dry naturally or blow dry and style as usual. (Recipe adapted from the "Wellness Mama" blog found here: wellnessmama.com)

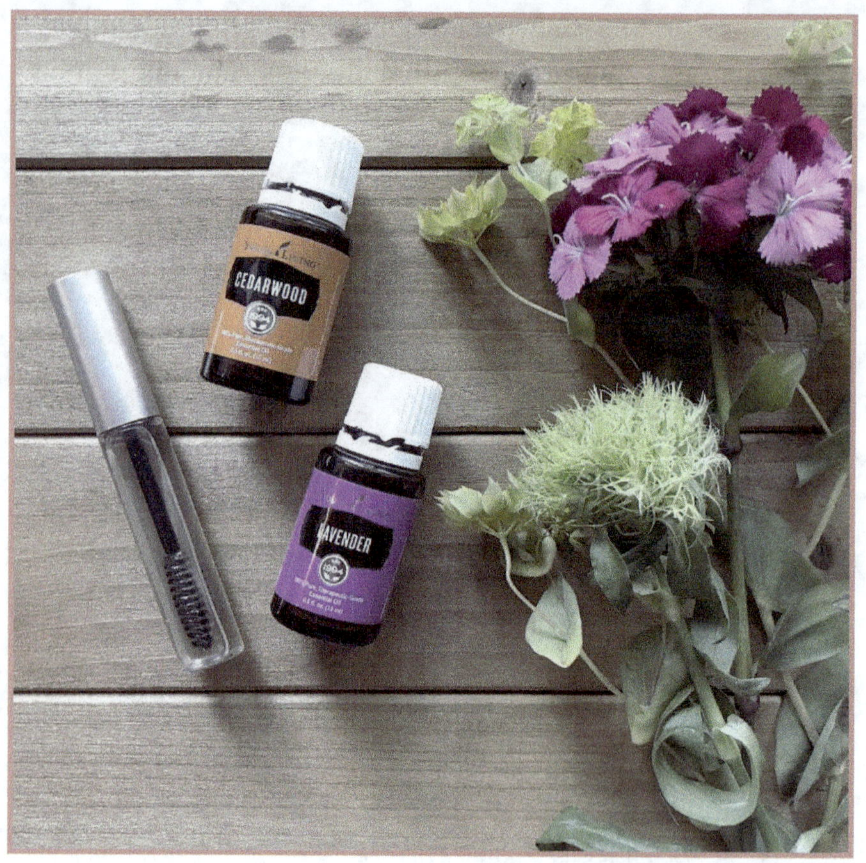

LASH BOOST SERUM

- o   Standard mascara tube
- o   10 drops Lavender
- o   10 drops Cedarwood
- o   5 drops Rosemary (optional)
- o   Castor oil

Add essential oil drops to the tube, then top with carrier oil. Gentle swirl around to incorporate. Apply to lashes at night, taking care to avoid direct contact with the eyes.

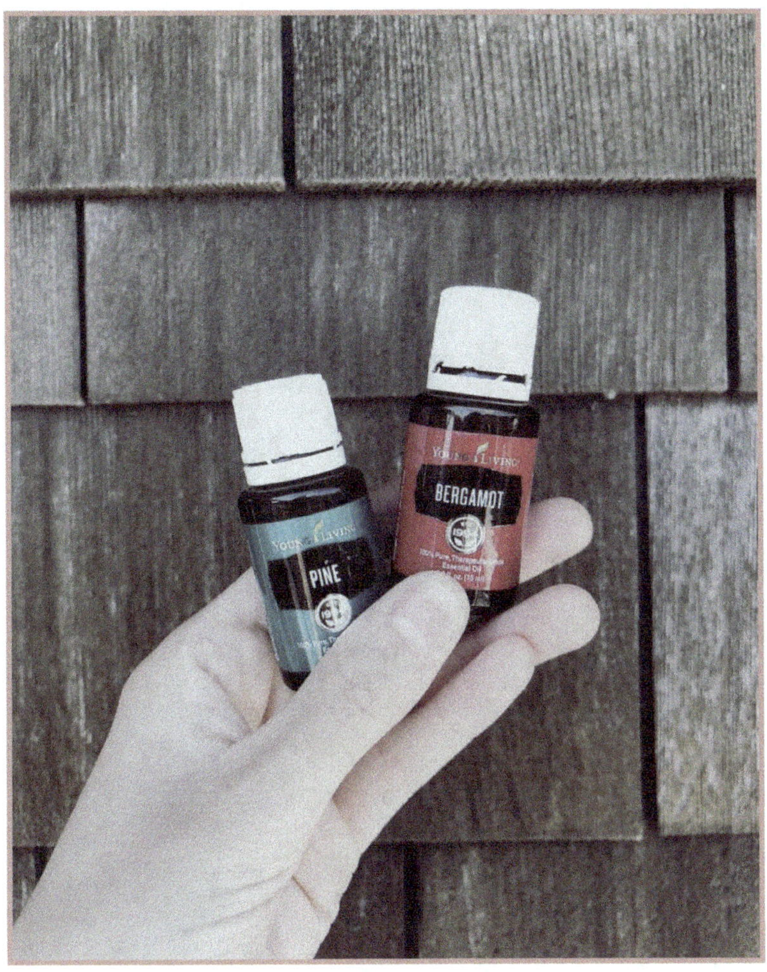

PINE & BERGAMOT FOAMING HAND SOAP

- o   Foaming soap dispenser bottle
- o   2 Tbsp. Dr. Bronner's Castile soap
- o   2 tsp. Fractionated coconut oil
- o   10 drops Pine
- o   10 drops Bergamot
- o   Distilled water

Combine all ingredients in the soap bottle and top with water. Shake well. Dispense 2-3 pumps of soap in palm, lather up, then rinse. Shake soap bottle every once in a while to incorporate ingredients. Try subbing essential oils for other such as Lavender and Eucalyptus or Christmas Spirit™.

CHILL OUT BATH SALT

- o   Bottle or jar with tight lid
- o   1 ½ cups Epsom salt
- o   ½ cup course sea salt (or Himalayan pink salt)
- o   ¼ cup baking soda
- o   12 drops Lavender
- o   12 drops Stress Away™
- o   Decoration such lavender petals (optional)

Place all ingredients in a bowl and mix together well.

These recipes are super practical and actually work. I hope you enjoy giving them a try!

STAIN SPRAY

- o   8 oz. glass spray bottle
- o   Thieves® laundry soap
- o   Thieves® household cleaner
- o   30 drops lemon
- o   Distilled water

Fill bottle 1/3 of the way with laundry soap. Add three capfuls of Thieves® cleaner, then add essential oil drops. Top with water. Shake well. Spray stained area until it's soaked through. Let sit for at least 20 minutes before throwing in the wash. (Recipe originally found on Instagram from Shelby Brunn: @wildflora. wellness)

LAUNDRY BRIGHTENER

- o   25 oz. glass bottle
- o   Thieves® household cleaner
- o   30 drops Lemon
- o   4 oz. hydrogen peroxide
- o   Distilled water

Add 2 capfuls of Thieves® cleaner, essential oil drops, and peroxide to the bottle. Top with water. Use a splash in each load. (Recipe originally found on Instagram from Shelby Brunn: @wildflora.wellness)

Tip: Reuse your Ningxia Red® bottles for recipes like this one!

SCENTED WOOL DRYER BALLS

Grab a pack of 6, 9, or 12 wool dryer balls from Amazon. They are very efficient and cost-effective, and they're natural! It's been said they can decrease drying time up to 25%. Dryer balls are the perfect way to ditch dryer sheets, which are known to be one of the most toxic household products. Just do a quick Google search on the toxicity of dryer sheets, and you'll definitely be wanting to replace them! Wool dryer balls last through 1,000 loads or about 5 to 8 years in the average house. You may be wondering, if I ditch my dryer sheets and switch to wool balls, how will my clothes smell wonderful, fresh and clean anymore? With this hack, they will! Lemongrass is my absolute favorite oil to use with wool dryer balls. I use 6 drops total for each load. Allow the oil to soak into the balls before tossing in the dryer with your laundry.

One thing having essential oils on hand is super convenient for is making supplements such as these as needed. It's like on-demand healthcare. Enjoy this collection of 4 supplement recipes!

TUMMY RESCUE SUPPLEMENT

- o   Veggie capsule size "0"
- o   4 drops Digize™ Vitality™
- o   2 drops Peppermint Vitality™
- o   Organic olive oil (or carrier oil of choice)

For each one, add essential oil drops to empty veggie capsule, and top with olive oil. Take twice a day, preferably morning and mid-afternoon. If you want to prepare in bulk, you can refrigerate them. Use within 2 weeks. Please note, if you do not use these as soon as they're prepared, capsules will begin to leek and disintegrate. Refrigeration helps delay this.

WEIGHT MANAGEMENT SUPPLEMENT

- o   Veggie capsule size "0"
- o   2-3 drops Lemon Vitality™
- o   2-3 drops Grapefruit Vitality™
- o   2-3 drops Peppermint Vitality™
- o   Organic olive oil (or carrier oil of choice)

For each one, add essential oil drops to empty veggie capsule, and top with olive oil. Take twice a day, morning and mid-afternoon. If you want to prepare in bulk, you can refrigerate them. Use within 2 weeks. Please note, if you do not use these as soon as they're prepared, capsules will begin to leek and disintegrate. Refrigeration helps delay this.

IMMUNE BOOSTER SUPPLEMENT

- o   Veggie capsule size "0"
- o   4 drops Thieves® Vitality™
- o   2 drops Oregano Vitality™
- o   2 drops Lemongrass Vitality™
- o   2 drops Frankincense Vitality™
- o   Organic olive oil (or carrier oil of choice)

For each one, add essential oil drops to empty veggie capsule, and top with olive oil. Take twice a day, morning and mid-afternoon. If you want to prepare in bulk, you can refrigerate them. Use within 2 weeks. Please note, if you do not use these as soon as they're prepared, capsules will begin to leek and disintegrate. Refrigeration helps delay this.

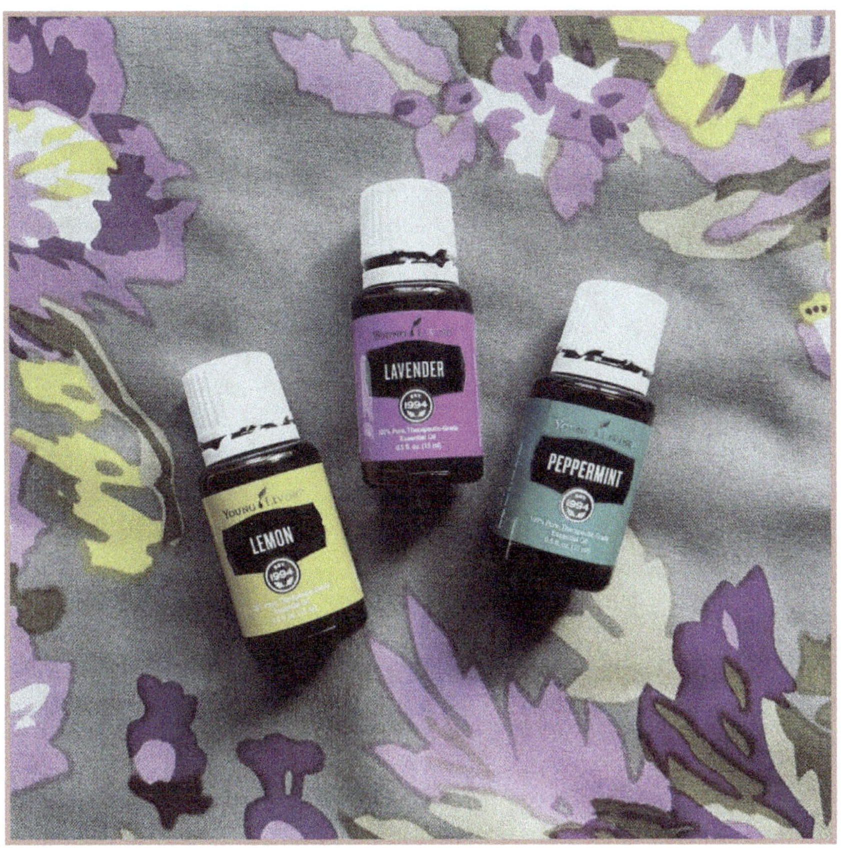

SEASONAL SUPPORT SUPPLEMENT

- o   Veggie capsule size "0"
- o   2-3 drops Lavender Vitality™
- o   2-3 drops Lemon Vitality™
- o   2-3 drops Peppermint Vitality™
- o   Organic olive oil (or carrier oil of choice)

For each one, add essential oil drops to empty veggie capsule, and top with olive oil. Take twice a day, preferably morning and mid-afternoon. If you want to prepare in bulk, you can refrigerate them. Use within 2 weeks. Please note, if you do not use these as soon as they're prepared, capsules will begin to leek and disintegrate. Refrigeration helps delay this.

Essential oils in food and drinks?! Yes, with Young Living's® Vitality™ line of oils, they can be safely consumed. Essential oils pack a powerful flavor punch! A little goes a long way. When one drop of oil is even too much, try the toothpick swirl method: Using a toothpick, lightly coat the tip with oil from the top of the bottle and then stir or swirl into the mixture. Enjoy this collection of 6 food and drink recipes. Cheers!

GUACAMOLE

serves 4-6

- o   3 large avocados, halved, seeded and peeled
- o   1/2 small onion, finely diced
- o   2 Roma tomatoes, diced
- o   1-2 garlic clove, minced
- o   1 lime, freshly juiced (or substitute with 2 drops of Lime Vitality™)
- o   ½ tsp. sea salt
- o   ¼ tsp. cayenne pepper
- o   1 drop Cumin Vitality™
- o   1 drop Cilantro Vitality™

In a medium bowl, mash the avocados making them as chunky or smooth as you'd like. Add lime juice and toss to coat. After all of the avocados have been coated, drain and reserve the lime juice. Mix in garlic, salt, cayenne, Cumin Vitality™ and Cilantro Vitality™. Then, fold in the onion and tomatoes. Add 1 tablespoon of the reserved lime juice. Garnish with cilantro (optional). Serve with chips.

VEGGIE CHICKEN SOUP

serves 10-12

- o   2 quarts chicken stock
- o   6 medium carrots
- o   2 large potatoes
- o   1 large onion
- o   1 ½ cups corn
- o   1 stalk celery, chopped
- o   8-1 0 brussel sprouts
- o   2 cups chicken
- o   2 tsp. salt
- o   1 tsp. pepper
- o   2 tsp. parsley flakes
- o   1 drop Rosemary Vitality™
- o   1 drop Oregano Vitality™
- o   1 drop Basil Vitality™
- o   1 drop Thyme Vitality™

Begin with a large soup pot. You can get chicken stock either from the store or try making your own by following a recipe such as this one:
cookingclassy.com/how-to-make-chicken-stock.

It's easy to make and a great way to use the leftover carcass from a rotisserie chicken. Peel and chop carrots into 1/4" thick pieces. Peel and cube potatoes. Chop onion and celery. Cut Brussel spouts in half. Prepare chicken into bite-size pieces. Once chicken stock is ready after being made or heated up, bring to a boil and add carrots and onion. Boil for about 10 minutes, then add potatoes and celery, boil for another 10 minutes and add the rest of the ingredients. Boil for 5 minutes, then simmer for 10. Add more chicken stock or water to get the right consistency if soup ends up too thick.

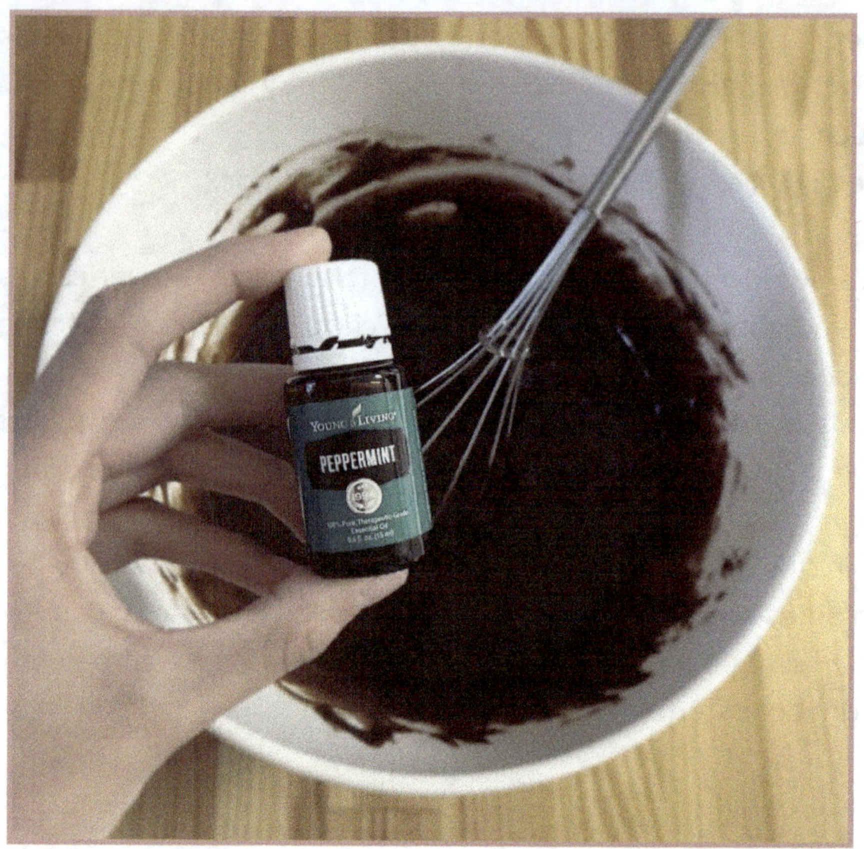

PEPPERMINT BROWNIES

serves 12

- o 1 brownie mix
- o Add 3 drops Peppermint Vitality™

Prepare standard brownie box mix or recipe. Add 3 drops Peppermint Vitality™ to the batter and thoroughly stir in. Bake normally.

LAVENDER LEMONADE

makes about 10 cups

- 6 lemons, juiced
- 1 lime, juiced
- ½ cup honey
- 2 drops Lavender Vitality™
- Ice water, about 10 cups
- Lavender sprigs, optional

Combine lemon juice, lime juice, honey, and Lavender Vitality™ in a large glass pitcher. Add water to taste. Stir until well mixed. Garnish with sprigs of lavender.

LAVENDER HOT CHOCOLATE

1 serving

- 1 cup unsweetened almond, dairy, or other milk of your choice
- 1 Tbsp. Cacao powder
- ¼ tsp. vanilla extract
- 1 Tbsp. honey, or more to taste
- 1 drop Lavender Vitality™

Heat milk in a saucepan on medium-high heat. Add 1 Tbsp. Cacao powder, 1/4 tsp. vanilla extract, and 1 Tbsp. honey; whisk until smooth. When warm, remove from heat and stir in 1 drop Lavender Vitality essential oil. Serve and enjoy!

EO INFUSED TEA

1 serving

- o   1 Tea bag (your choice)
- o   1 drop Thieves® Vitality™
- o   1 drop Lemon Vitality™
- o   1 tsp. Honey

Drop oils directly onto tea bag. Make tea as usual.

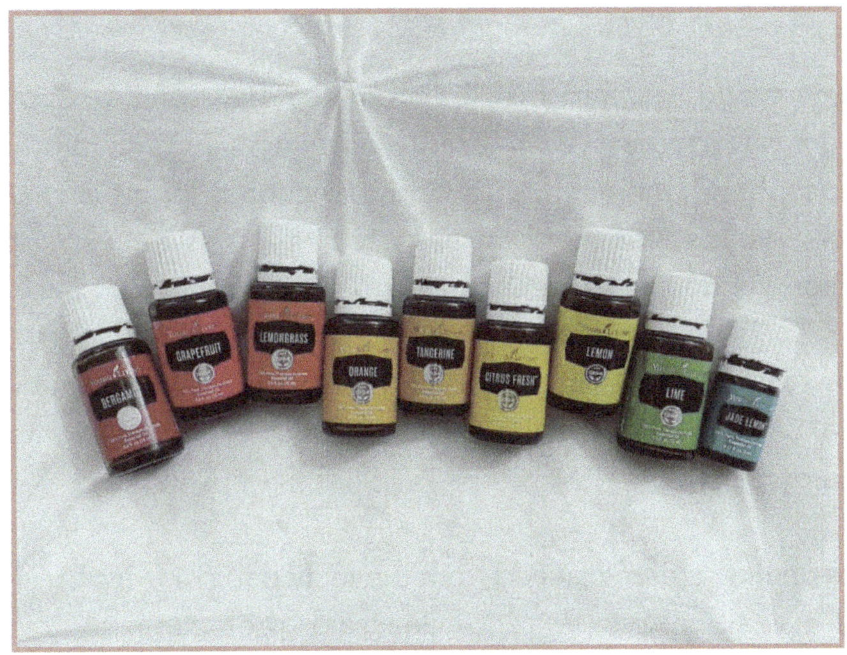

Curious about the oils used in these recipes? Here's a little info on each:

Believe™ - a blend of Balsam Canada, Coriander, Bergamot, Frankincense, Idaho Blue Spruce, Ylang Ylang and Geranium; may promote feelings of strength and faith

Bergamot - cold pressed from the yellow-green peel of an orange-shaped citrus fruit; known for its mood-lifting, cleansing and calming qualities

Blue Tansy - harvested from tiny yellow flowers in the chamomile family, the naturally occurring constituent chamazulene turns the powerfully pure Blue Tansy essential oil a beautifully rich blue color during the steam distillation process; known for its relaxing, cleansing, muscle soothing, and calming benefits; also great for the skin

Cedarwood - steam distilled from the bark of the *Cedrus atlantica*; creates a relaxing, calming and comforting atmosphere when diffused; body function support includes the nervous system, respiratory system, skin, tissue, hair, limbic system, endocrine system and sleep

Christmas Spirit™ - an invigorating blend of Orange, Cinnamon and Black Spruce; has purifying qualities and may promote energy balance

Citronella - steam distilled from the leafy parts of the citronella plant; may provide relaxing, cleansing, protecting, soothing, freshening, critter repelling and muscle calming benefits

Citrus Fresh™ - an uplifting blend of Orange, Tangerine, Grapefruit, Lemon, Mandarin and Spearmint; known for its energizing and purifying qualities; may promote mental clarity

Copaiba - a product of steam distilling the gum resin tapped from the Brazilian *Copaifera reticulata* tree; body function support includes emotional balance, respiratory system, muscles, skin, circulatory system and nervous system

Cypress - has a fresh, herbaceous aroma that can promote a sense of security and grounding; body function support includes the respiratory system, nervous system, immune system, circulatory system, and muscles/joints/bones

Eucalyptus Radiata - steam distilled from the leaves of the *Eucalyptus radiata* tree; known for its cleansing, clearing and soothing benefits; body function support includes the respiratory system, circulatory system and skin

Frankincense - steam distilled from the resin of *Boswellia carterii* tree; may provide cleansing, protecting, calming, soothing, regenerative, muscle calming and emotional supporting benefits

Gentle Baby™ - a soothing blend of Coriander, Geranium, Palmarosa, Lavender, Ylang Ylang, Roman Chamomile, Bergamot, Lemon, Jasmine and Rose; invites a sense of calm; perfect for diffusing at night to promote rest and relaxation

Geranium - steam distilled from the flowers and leaves of the *Pelargonium graveolens* plant; may provide stimulating, cleansing, protecting, revitalizing, uplifting, regenerative and muscle calming benefits

Grounding™ - a unique combination of White Fir, Northern Lights Black Spruce, Ylang Ylang, Pine, Cedarwood, Angelica and Juniper; may provide stress relief, mental clarity and emotional balance

Helichrysum - steam distilled from the blossoms of *Helichrysum italicum*; known for its cleansing, protecting, regenerative, dissolving, stimulating, balancing and flushing properties

Joy™ - a delightful blend of Bergamot, Ylang Ylang, Geranium, Lemon, Coriander, Tangerine, Jasmine, Roman Chamomile, Palmarosa and Rose; may support emotional balance and elevated mood

Lavender - steam distilled from the flowering tops of the *Lavandula angustifolia* plant; therapeutic effects may include calming, soothing, muscle calming, emotional support, relaxing, cleansing, protecting, renewing and regenerating; body function support includes skin, digestion, the respiratory system, tissue, blood, nervous system, emotions, limbic system, endocrine system, hormones, nerves, wound support and sleep

Lemon - cold pressed from the rind of lemons; 75 lemons are required to make one 15ml bottle of Lemon essential oil; therapeutic effects may include cleansing, flushing, calming, uplifting, and clarification; body function support includes the circulatory system, respiratory system, skin, digestion and emotions

Lemongrass - steam distilled from the grassy part of the *Cymbopogon flexuosus* plant; may provide cleansing, calming, regenerative, purifying, and protecting benefits

Lime - cold pressed from the rind of limes; body function support includes the respiratory system, immune system, skin, lymphatic system and emotions

Northern Lights Black Spruce - every part of the tree is used to produce this oil; therapeutic effects may include grounding, relieving, flushing, relaxing, balancing and revitalizing; body function support includes the immune system, endocrine system, hormones, sleep, respiratory system and sleep

Orange - cold pressed from the rind of oranges; therapeutic effects may include uplifting, calming, cleansing, repairing and soothing; body function support includes the respiratory system, circulatory system, digestion, sleep, hormones, muscles/bones, tissue and skin

Panaway™ - a blend of Wintergreen, Helichrysum, Clove and Peppermint; body function support includes muscle soothing, cooling and stimulating

Peace & Calming® - a blend of Tangerine, Orange, Ylang Ylang, Patchouli and Blue Tansy; can help create a calm, comforting environment; may help relieve stress, anxiety and tension

Peppermint - steam distilled from peppermint leaves; body function support includes the respiratory system, circulatory system, digestion, skin, muscles, bones, focus and energy

Pine - therapeutic effects may include protecting, cleansing, stimulating, relieving, empowering and grounding; body function support includes the respiratory system, hormones, mind, emotions and skin

Purification® - a blend of Citronella, Rosemary, Lemongrass, Tea Tree, Lavandin and Myrtle; acts as a powerful air freshener by cleaning and purifying the air; eliminates bad odors

Rosemary - steam distilled from the *Rosmarinus officinalis*, a perennial shrub; has a robust, herbaceous aroma; body function support includes muscles, liver, mental, emotions and immunity

Sacred Frankincense - comes from the distillation of the resin of the *Boswellia sacra* frankincense tree; body function support includes joints, tendons, muscles, the limbic system, endocrine system, respiratory system, circulatory system, nervous system and emotions; may provide calming, cleansing, protective, regenerative and soothing benefits

Seedlings® Calm™ - a gentle blend of Lavender, Coriander, Bergamot, Ylang Ylang and Geranium; therapeutic effects include relaxing and calming

Spearmint - steam distilled from spearmint leaves; milder than peppermint and characterized by stimulating, balancing, uplifting, soothing and invigorating benefits

Stress Away™ - a blend of Copaiba, Lime, Cedarwood, Vanilla Extract, Ocotea and Lavender; its unique and pleasant aroma is relaxing and comforting; may promote stress relief, relaxation, focus and sleep

Thieves® - a powerful blend of Clove, Lemon, Cinnamon Bark, Eucalyptus Radiata and Rosemary known for its purifying qualities and for supporting proper immune function

Valor® - a blend of Caprylic/Capric Triglyceride, Northern Lights Black Spruce, Camphor, Blue Tansy, Frankincense and Geranium; may provide grounding, energy and balance; may promote feelings of courage, empowerment and confidence

Vetiver - steam distilled from the root of the *Vetiveria zizanoides* plant; has a deep, earthy woodsy scent; may provide grounding, calming, stabilizing and relaxing benefits; may promote a feeling of protection

White Angelica™ - a blend of Sweet Almond Oil, Bergamot, Myrrh, Geranium, Sandalwood, Ylang Ylang, Coriander, Northern Lights Black Spruce, Melissa, Hyssop and Rose; has a lovely rounded aroma with the combination of floral, citrus and woodsy oils; may promote feelings of protection and security; also has skin-beautifying benefits

INTERNAL-USE OILS

Basil Vitality™ - steam distilled from the leaves of the *Ocimum basilicum* plant; has a sweet, warm scent and flavor; body function support includes the circulatory system, muscles, bones, immune system and respiratory system

Cilantro Vitality™ - steam distilled from the *Coriandrum sativum* plant; body function support includes the immune system, digestion, and internal cleansing

Cumin Vitality™ - comes from the seeds of the *Cuminum cyminum* plant; delivers internal cleansing properties and provides support for the body's most important detoxifying organs, like the liver, kidneys, and digestive system

Digize™ Vitality™ - a blend consisting of Tarragon, Ginger, Peppermint, Juniper, Fennel, Lemongrass, Anise and Patchouli; provides support to the digestive system

Frankincense Vitality™ - steam distilled from the resin of *Boswellia carterii* tree; body function support includes the limbic system, endocrine system, respiratory system, circulatory system, nervous system and emotions

Grapefruit Vitality™ - cold pressed from the rind of grapefruits; may provide cleansing, flushing and uplifting benefits; body function support includes digestion, tissue, skin, fat cells, lymphatic system, kidney, liver and emotions

Lavender Vitality™ - steam distilled from the flowering tops of the *Lavandula angustifolia* plant; therapeutic effects may include calming, soothing, muscle calming, emotional support, relaxing, cleansing, protecting, renewing and regenerating; body function support includes skin, digestion, the respiratory system, tissue, blood, nervous system, emotions, limbic system, endocrine system, hormones, nerves, wound support and sleep

Lemon Vitality™ - cold pressed from the rind of lemons; 75 lemons are required to make one 15ml bottle of Lemon essential oil; therapeutic effects may include cleansing, flushing, calming, uplifting, and clarification; body function support includes the circulatory system, respiratory system, skin, digestion and emotions

Lemongrass Vitality™ - steam distilled from the grassy part of the *Cymbopogon flexuosus* plant; may provide cleansing, calming, regenerative, purifying, and protecting benefits

Lime Vitality™ - cold pressed from the rind of limes; body function support includes the respiratory system, immune system, skin, lymphatic system and emotions

Oregano Vitality™ - comes from the *Origanum vulgare* plant; body function support includes the respiratory system, circulatory system, and lymphatic system; may provide cleansing, flushing and strengthening benefits

Peppermint Vitality™ - steam distilled from peppermint leaves; body function support includes the respiratory system, circulatory system, digestion, skin, muscles, bones, focus and energy

Rosemary Vitality™ - steam distilled from the *Rosmarinus officinalis*, a perennial shrub; has a robust, herbaceous aroma; body function support includes muscles, liver, mental, emotions and immunity

Thieves® Vitality™ - a powerful blend of Clove, Lemon, Cinnamon Bark, Eucalyptus Radiata and Rosemary known for its purifying qualities and for supporting proper immune function

Thyme Vitality™ - steam distilled from the leaves of the *Thymus vulgaris* plant; may provide cleansing, soothing, protecting, purifying and energizing benefits to the body

LINKS TO SUPPLIES

Besides the oils themselves, there are a number of supplies and materials, such as roller bottles, diffusers and carrier oils, nice to have on hand for making these recipes. The good news is many of the recipes use a lot of the same ingredients-for example fractionated coconut oil and witch hazel. Make sure to check out my Amazon storefront for links to my favorites! I've curated my Amazon recommendations to help you out by making it like a one-stop-shop for these supplies. I've also linked to several shops where you can find cute essential oil accessories.

MY AMAZON FINDS

amazon.com/shop/joyful.and.well

LINKS TO SHOPS WITH CUTE OIL BAGS AND OTHER ACCESSORIES

modernmakerie.com
whimsyandwellness.com
etsy.com/shop/BaggageandCO
etsy.com/shop/PineAndPouch
etsy.com/shop/TuckerDesignCompany

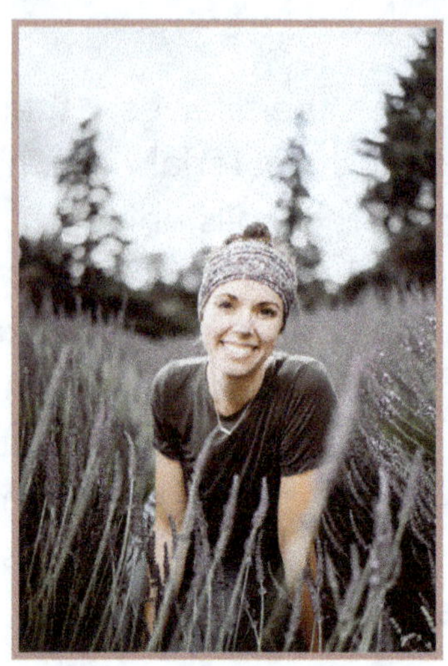

Alexis fell in love with essential oils in 2017 and has been using them in the pursuit of wellness ever since. She is an occasional writer, full-time business owner and board-certified music therapist. She loves hiking, reading, traveling, inspiring quotes, music, health and wellness, personal development, Jesus and connecting with people. Alexis lives in Portland, OR with her husband Tom. You can connect with her on Instagram (@joyful.and.well) or reach out via email: **Alexis@joyfulandwell.com**

Her Young Living® referral ID is 11400891

www.ingramcontent.com/pod-product-compliance
Lightning Source LLC
Chambersburg PA
CBHW060801260726

48660CB00002B/719